What Every Speech Language Pathologist/Audiologist Should Know About Augmentative and Alternative Communication

Jennifer Kent-Walsh
University of Central Florida

Cathy Binger
University of New Mexico

Boston Columbus Indianapolis New York San Francisco Upper Saddle River

Amsterdam Cape Town Dubai London Madrid Milan Munich Paris Montreal Toronto

Delhi Mexico City Sao Paulo Sydney Hong Kong Seoul Singapore Taipei Tokyo

Printed in the United States of America

10 9 8 7 6 5 4   V013   15 14 13 12

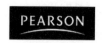

ISBN-10: 0-13-706881-6
ISBN-13: 978-0-13-706881-4

www.pearsonhighered.com

CONTENTS

ABOUT THE AUTHORS

Cathy Binger, Ph.D., CCC-SLP, is an assistant professor in the Department of Speech and Hearing Sciences at the University of New Mexico. In addition to teaching undergraduate and graduate courses in speech-language pathology, Cathy conducts research in AAC in conjunction with her research partner, Jennifer Kent-Walsh. Cathy's main area of research interest is in developing and evaluating intervention programs to improve language and communication outcomes for children who use AAC.

Jennifer Kent-Walsh, Ph.D., CCC-SLP, S-LP(C), is an Associate Professor in the Department of Communication Sciences and Disorders at the University of Central Florida. In addition to conducting AAC-related research and teaching undergraduate and graduate courses in AAC and language, Jennifer is the Director of the Florida Alliance for Assistive Services and Technology (FAAST) Atlantic Region Assistive Technology Demonstration Center.

ACKNOWLEDGEMENTS

The authors would like to extend their sincere thanks to the many clients and families who have illustrated the power and potential of AAC to them over the years and to the many students who have expressed such keen interest in being introduced to the field of AAC. Special thanks also go out to Stephanie McDougle and Jennifer Moss for their assistance in the preparation of this book.

CHAPTER 1

What is AAC?

Introduction

This book is all about augmentative and alternative communication (AAC), which is an area of practice that has become central to the field of speech-language pathology (SLP). To help you gain a thorough understanding of AAC, we will talk in this chapter about: (a) what AAC is, (b) who can benefit from the use of AAC, (c) what kinds of AAC solutions are available for people, and (d) when and where AAC might be useful to people.

Given your interest in the field of SLP, you may have some prior knowledge of AAC. Let's begin by seeing if you have any ideas about the types of clients who could benefit from AAC. Can you determine which of the following clients might benefit from the use of some form of AAC?

- A **child in the fifth grade** has **cerebral palsy**. She uses a wheelchair for mobility, and her speech is extremely hard to understand. She understands everything that is said to her, including all directions and instructions for her school work, but she does not have the motor skills necessary to speak clearly or to write. She uses specialized software on the classroom computer that she uses to complete her school work.

- A **preschooler, age three,** has just been diagnosed with an **autism spectrum disorder**. He uses a few words to talk, but the words do not always seem relevant for a given situation. For example, he often says "Pickles!" when he walks into the preschool room, even though the children have never eaten pickles at school. He follows some simple directions, but the only way he asks for what he wants is by picking up objects. He demonstrates rejection by throwing

1

items, pushing items away, or getting up and leaving an unwanted situation.

- A **17-year-old student** with **Down syndrome** uses his speech to communicate. His family and close friends understand what he says a lot of the time, especially when they have some context for the conversation – for example, if they know he's telling them something about a ski vacation. It is harder for unfamiliar people to understand him, but he is persistent and will keep trying to make himself understood by repeating himself again and again.

- A **young adult on the autism spectrum** is considered "high functioning." She uses her speech and language appropriately in many situations, and she speaks in full sentences. She comprehends what is said to her, as long as the information is fairly concrete. She has a phenomenal memory for places she has been and can draw them in great detail. She can become agitated, however, when she goes to new places and is introduced to new things, such as taking a trip to a museum for the first time or visiting a new doctor's office.

- A **22 year old man** has a **traumatic brain injury** (TBI) resulting from a motor cycle accident; he was not wearing a helmet. His speech is extremely slurred and hard to understand, but he can speak in full sentences. He understands concrete messages, but has a harder time with more abstract topics of conversation, such as discussions about current political events.

- A **49-year-old woman** has recently been diagnosed with **amyotrophic lateral sclerosis** (ALS, also known as Lou Gehrig's disease). Right now, her speech and language skills are fine. The only symptoms she currently has are weakness in her arms and legs.

- A **65 year old man** recently had a **stroke** that affected his speech and language. He can say some words clearly, although they are not always the words he means to say. He knows what he wants to say, but he has severe word-finding problems and uses telegraphic speech. He also uses lots of gestures, pantomime, and drawings to help get his point across. He understands nearly all of what others say to him.

- An **elderly woman** is in a nursing home and has **dementia**. Her memory is worsening, but she is able to share memories of past events with photo albums, which she enjoys tremendously. During such discussions, she becomes very animated. She is starting to have some swallowing problems and is receiving SLP services to make sure she is safe while eating and drinking.

So, what do you think – which of the above people might benefit from using AAC, and which people are doing just fine without AAC? The fact is, *all* of the people in the above scenarios could potentially benefit from using AAC, and many of them already *are* using AAC. Although these people demonstrate very different abilities and disabilities, they all have at least one thing in common: none of them is able to communicate and/or participate in daily activities to their maximum ability without the help of AAC. Later in this chapter, we will revisit these cases to see what types of AAC each person is using or could potentially benefit from using. However, we need to examine exactly what AAC is first. We also need to consider the related category of assistive technology (AT).

What is AAC? What is AT?

First, let's look at the first two words within the term "AAC." 'Augment' implies a form of supplementation and 'alternative' implies a form of replacement. AAC, then, means using some form of communication that is designed to either supplement or replace more typical means of communication. Frequently, this means using something other than speech to communicate. For example, the three year old with autism described in the previous section may learn to use a photograph or line drawing of a pretzel (instead of the spoken word "pretzel") to tell his father that he wants a pretzel or to tell his mother that he had pretzels for a snack. Another example of using photographs can be found in the previous example of the woman with dementia; she is supplementing communication by using photographs to share information about her life

3

and to provide topics of conversation. Another example of AAC use can be found in the previous example of the gentleman who had a stroke. Before his stroke, he used his speech to communicate; now, he is supplementing his speech by also making extensive use of other forms of communication, including gestures, pantomime, and drawings. All of these forms of communication – line drawings, photographs, gestures, pantomime – are forms of AAC.

The American Speech-Language-Hearing Association, or ASHA (2005), which is the professional, scientific, and credentialing association for audiologists, speech-language pathologists and related scientists in the United States, provides the following definition of AAC:

> *Augmentative and alternative communication (AAC) refers to an area of research, clinical, and educational practice. AAC involves attempts to study and when necessary compensate for temporary or permanent impairments, activity limitations, and participation restrictions of individuals with severe disorders of speech-language production and/or comprehension, including spoken and written modes of communication* (p. 413).

Let's take a moment to examine each component of this definition.

1. First, it is important to note that AAC involves research, clinical, and educational practice. That means that AAC can be used in a wide range of settings, including research settings such as within universities, clinical settings such as hospitals, nursing homes, or private practices, and educational settings, including all school environments. AAC, then, is used across a very wide range of settings.

2. Next, the definition indicates that AAC can be used with people who have either temporary or permanent impairments. An example of a temporary impairment would be someone who has a tube put in their airway (that is, a tracheotomy) so that they can breathe, and this tube may remain in place for a period of time following

surgery. In contrast, all of the cases presented earlier in this chapter are examples of permanent impairments.

3. People who have communication disorders may experience activity limitations or participation restrictions as a result of their impairments. For example, all of the children in a preschool classroom may take turns stating what the weather is like, except for one child who has no intelligible speech. Or a person who has a communication disorder resulting from a stroke may no longer participate in a weekly poker game with their friends. In both cases, someone is not fully participating in their daily activities due to a communication disorder. AAC may play an important role in allowing people to participate more fully in these types of everyday activities.

4. AAC solutions may be appropriate for people who have speech as well as language impairments. For example, in the previously discussed examples, the man with TBI primarily has a speech impairment – he has slurred speech but can still speak in full sentences – and the child with autism, who has little functional vocabulary and is not creating sentences at all, is exhibiting a significant language impairment (which may also be accompanied by a speech impairment).

5. Also, AAC can be used to promote not only expressive communication (i.e., production), but also receptive communication (i.e., comprehension). The three-year-old with autism may use photographs and line drawings to request objects (such as pretzels), which is a form of production. In addition, his teachers may have visual schedules set up in his classroom containing series of line drawings to help him understand what is expected of him. For example, his visual schedule by the classroom door may contain drawings representing each of the major tasks of the day, such as circle time, snack time, and an art activity. The young woman with autism described in the previous examples may benefit from a similar type of tool called a "social story" (Sansosti, 2004), in

which a series of line drawings or photos of what she might encounter at the museum or the doctor's office are depicted.

6. Finally, AAC includes the use of both spoken and written communication modes. In today's world, most individuals spend time each day engaged not only in spoken communication (whether face-to-face or via telecommunications) but also in various forms of written communication, including activities such as sending e-mail and text messages (a form of language production) and reading e-mail and text messages (which involves comprehension).

AAC, then, can be used by people who have an extraordinary range of disabilities within a wide range of contexts. Communication takes place within all aspects of our lives and, according to ASHA (2005), "Communication is the essence of human life." ASHA also maintains that "all people have the right to communicate to the fullest extent possible. No individuals should be denied this right, irrespective of the type and/or severity of communication, linguistic, social, cognitive, motor, sensory, perceptual, and/or other disability(ies) they may present."

AAC is related to assistive technology, or AT. As discussed above, AAC refers to communication solutions for people with various types of communication disorders. AT is defined as "any item, piece of equipment, or product system, whether acquired commercially, off the shelf, modified, or customized, that is used to increase, maintain, or improve the functional capabilities of individuals with disabilities" (Tech Act, 1988). In other words, AT is a broad category which includes any type of technology that a person might use to compensate for an impairment, such as using a wheelchair, walker, or communication device. In contrast, AAC only refers to solutions that focus on improving communication skills. AT is *not*, however, an umbrella term that encompasses AAC; AAC includes communication solutions which are not considered types of AT, such as the use of gestures and manual signs. Rather, AAC and AT are terms that overlap to some degree (for example, a computerized voice output device is both a form of AAC and AT), but both include components that do not overlap.

Communication Bill of Rights

To help ensure that all people have the right to communicate to the fullest extent possible, the National Joint Committee for the Communication Needs of Persons with Severe Disabilities (1992) developed a Communication Bill of Rights. The bill stipulates that all people are entitled to the following communication rights in their daily interactions:

- To request desired objects, actions, events and people
- To refuse undesired objects, actions, or events
- To express personal preferences and feelings
- To be offered choices and alternatives
- To reject offered choices
- To request and receive another person's attention and interaction
- To ask for and receive information about changes in routine and environment
- To receive intervention to improve communication skills
- To receive a response to any communication, whether or not the responder can fulfill the request
- To have access to AAC (augmentative and alternative communication) and other AT (assistive technology) services and devices at all times
- To have AAC and other AT devices that function properly at all times
- To be in environments that promote one's communication as a full partner with other people, including peers
- To be spoken to with respect and courtesy
- To be spoken to directly and not be spoken for or talked about in the third person while present
- To have clear, meaningful and culturally and linguistically appropriate communications

Everyone, then – regardless of type or severity of their disabilities – is entitled to appropriate means of communication and to enjoy the same basic respect enjoyed by people who do not have communication disorders. We are sure that this basic premise is something on which we can all agree!

Who Needs AAC?

Which individuals, exactly, might benefit from using AAC? In the previous examples, there are individuals with a wide range of disabilities across a wide range of ages – in fact, across the entire lifespan – all of whom can benefit from using AAC. Regardless of the type of disability, all people who use AAC have one thing in common: their communication and participation needs are not met by the use of speech alone. In many cases, this means the person needs to use another form of communication to express themselves. In other cases, AAC may be used help someone organize their world to increase participation, such as when someone uses a visual schedule or a social story, as described above. AAC also might be used to improve comprehension; for example, someone who has aphasia, a condition often caused by strokes that can affect language comprehension, might benefit from having the speaker write down key words as they are talking to help the person with aphasia understand the conversation better, as well as enable the person to make choices (Beukelman, 2005).

As you probably know, broadly speaking, there are two main types of communication disorders: developmental and acquired. People who have developmental disabilities are still in the process of developing their initial language skills and are not yet adults. Many people with developmental disorders have congenital disorders; that is, they were born with some type of disability, such as cerebral palsy or Down syndrome. In contrast, people with acquired disorders developed language typically for a period of time, but then experienced some type of trauma, such as a traumatic brain injury, stroke, or brain tumor, which resulted in a communication disorder. Table 1.1 lists common developmental and acquired communication disorders which may result in the need for AAC interventions. These interventions may differ markedly for a person with a developmental disorder versus and individual with an acquired disorder. For example, a child with a developmental disorder may need AAC to assist with learning basic language skills, such as how to put words of a sentence together for the first time, whereas an adult with a traumatic brain injury or stroke may have very slurred speech (dysarthria) but have language skills that are fully intact, and only need AAC to clarify messages that are not understood.

Table 1-1

Examples of Developmental and Acquired Disorders
Which Can Result in AAC Needs

Developmental Disorders	Acquired Disorders
Autism spectrum disorders	Amyotrophic lateral sclerosis
Cerebral palsy	Brain tumor
Childhood apraxia of speech	Dementia
Cognitive impairment/ Intellectual disability	Guillain-Barré syndrome
Infectious diseases (e.g., maternal rubella)	Multiple sclerosis
Spina bifida	Parkinson's disease
Syndromes (e.g., Cornelia de Lange, Down syndrome)	Spinal cord injury
	Stroke
	Traumatic brain injury (TBI)

Each type of disorder listed in Table 1.1 also can be classified as progressive (also called "degenerative") or non-progressive. Most of the disorders in Table 1.1 are non-progressive; that is, these conditions are relatively stable over time, or they may improve. For example, following a stroke, many people go through a period of spontaneous recovery in which some lost functioning may be recovered. In contrast, ALS and dementia are both progressive disorders; individuals with these disorders will experience deterioration of various functions over time, including speech and/or language skills.

It is also important to note the wide range of physical abilities of people who can benefit from the use of AAC. Some people may have no physical disabilities at all, such as some individuals with CAS or TBI. Commonly,

9

however, people using AAC also have some degree of physical impairment, from mild to profound. It is common, for example, for people who have aphasia resulting from a stroke to have weakness in their right arms and legs. Some people with cerebral palsy, as well as other impairments such as Locked-In Syndrome (caused by strokes), have profound physical impairments that significantly limit their independent mobility. In addition to having mobility impairments, many of these same individuals also have dysphagia, or swallowing disorders, which are treated by speech-language pathologists as well. When working with individuals who need AAC, physical capabilities must be carefully assessed in order to find AAC solutions that maximize use of residual physical capabilities.

What AAC Options are Available?

So far, we have talked about how AAC is defined and some people who may benefit from AAC, but what does AAC really look like? What types of AAC solutions are possible? Before we can discuss the wide range of AAC options, we must first discuss the terminology that is used to describe different types of AAC. First, we will discuss three different ways to categorize AAC options.

1. *Unaided versus aided*: All types of AAC can be broken down into two broad areas: *unaided* versus *aided* AAC. Unaided AAC includes the use of only the body to communicate, without external equipment of any kind. Gestures, manual signs, pantomime, gaze, vocalizations (which can convey emotional states or can approximate words), and head nods/shakes are all forms of unaided AAC. In contrast, aided AAC involves some type of external equipment, however simple or complex it may be; this category includes everything from a photograph of a glass of juice to represent *thirsty* to a computerized voice output device that says *THIRSTY* when you press a designated button.

2. *No tech versus low/mid tech versus high tech*: Aided AAC can be further broken down into *no tech, low tech*, and *high tech* types of devices. Different people define these terms in slightly different

ways. For our purposes, we will use the term *no tech* to refer to refer to any type of aided AAC that is non-electronic; that is, if it doesn't use a battery and you can't plug it in, it's a form of "no tech" aided AAC. *Low/mid tech* refers to simple electronic devices, typically those that do not have built-in rechargeable batteries, and record and play back a limited number of messages. *High tech* devices include the more expensive electronic devices, many of which can be purchased as fully functional computers.

3. *Dedicated versus. non-dedicated speech-generating devices*: All AAC devices also can be classified as either *dedicated* or *non-dedicated* devices. Dedicated devices, also known as *speech-generating devices (SGDs)*, are used solely for the purpose of speech generation. Typically, their primary function is to enhance communication during face-to-face interactions. These include both low/mid tech and high tech communication options. In contrast, non-dedicated devices are usually fully functioning computers that can run software programs that do more than generate speech. For example, a person using a non-dedicated device can typically access the Internet and load any type of software onto the hard drive of the device, such as word processing, email, or gaming software, just as a person would do with any other type of computer. Many AAC device manufacturers modify fully functioning computers to act as AAC devices, and oddly enough, they may "lock out" the regular computer functions, so that the device may be sold as an SGD. This happens despite the fact that the client who will be using the device may also need access to other computer functions, including all of the communication-based reasons for which you use a computer: for example, conducting research for a class project, writing class assignments, sharing information via Facebook™, or emailing friends and family. The reason behind this phenomenon is that most insurance companies in the United States (at least, as of this time) will not pay for fully functioning computers for people who need AAC; they will only pay for SGDs. Although this is an improvement over the days when many insurance companies did

not pay for AAC devices, it is nevertheless problematic for people who use AAC. Communication needs exist far beyond face-to-face, and being able to use electronic media for a wide array of purposes is essential communication in today's world.

To review, then, AAC can be classified as aided or unaided. Aided AAC can be further categorized as no, low/mid or high tech, and as dedicated or non-dedicated. In addition, we also need to discuss the different types of aided symbols that a person may use; that is, the way messages are represented on an AAC device. Table 1.2 lists some commonly used aided AAC symbols and provides examples of each type. Some of these symbols, such as real, partial, and miniature objects, typically are used only as part of no tech AAC. Others, such as photographs, line drawings, and written words (i.e., orthography) frequently are used as no, low/mid and high tech AAC.

Table 1-2

Various Types of Aided AAC Symbols and Examples of How They are Used

Aided AAC Symbol	Example
Real object	A spoon to represent *hungry*
Partial object	A guitar string to represent *music*
Miniature object	A small, plastic house to represent *home*
Photograph	A photograph of Dad to represent *Dad*
Line drawing	A drawing of carrots to represent *carrots*
Logo	A drawing of the Golden Arches to represent a McDonald's™ restaurant
Orthography (e.g., written/ typed letters, Braille, fingerspelling)	A keyboard is used to spell words, which are then spoken by a speech synthesizer on a computer; Braille and fingerspelling are used to represent each letter of the alphabet

Now that we have discussed some of the background information, we can discuss aided AAC devices themselves. The "containers" that house AAC devices vary dramatically and are chosen for any given person based on his individualized needs and preferences – for example, one person may need to use individually laminated symbols, and someone else may use a computerized communication device. Similarly, one person may prefer to have a pink computer or communication device, whereas another individual may prefer a black communication device. Table 1.3 lists some of the types of aided AAC devices that are available. In addition to variance across the categories we just discussed (no versus low/mid versus high tech, dedicated versus non-dedicated, types of symbols available), devices vary in a number of additional ways, including the following:

1. number of symbols
2. spacing of symbols
3. size of symbols
4. size of container
5. overall portability (size, weight, handle, etc.)
6. durability
7. availability of electronic functions like environmental controls (e.g., able to operate TV/VCR), infrared options (e.g., for a printer), and telephone access
8. type of display: static versus dynamic
   a. static = unchanging, such as any paper-based display
   b. dynamic = changing based on user input, such as an electronic computer screen or ATM machine screen)
9. access method: direct selection versus scanning
   a. direct selection = the user touches, points to, looks at, or in some other way directly makes a choice
   b. scanning = someone or something else is "offers" choices; person using AAC indicates when the desired item is offered

Table 1-3   Various Types of Aided AAC Devices

Aided AAC Device Characteristics	Type of Symbol Used	No, Low or High Tech?	Static/ Dynamic Display	Examples
Single symbols (usually laminated)[1]	Line drawings or photos	No tech	static	
Communication album/board/ book/ wallet[2]	Line drawings, photos, logos, orthography	No tech	static	

14

Table 1-3 Continued Various Types of Aided AAC Devices

Aided AAC Device	Type of Symbol	No, Low or High	Static/ Dynamic	Examples
Remnant book or pocket[3]	Movie tickets, brochures, menus, etc.	No tech	static	
Gaze board (usually plexiglass)[4]	Line drawings or photos	No tech	static	

Table 1-3 Continued   Various Types of Aided AAC Devices

Aided AAC Device Characterist	Type of Symbol Used	No, Low or High Tech?	Static/Dynamic Display	Examples
Single message SGD[5]	Line drawings or photos	Line drawings or photos	static	
Multi-symbol SGD (static display)[6,]	Line drawings, photos, logos	Low or high tech	Static	

Table 1-3 Continued   Various Types of Aided AAC Devices

Aided AAC Device Characteristics	Type of Symbol Used	No, Low or High Tech?	Static/ Dynamic Display	Examples
Multi-symbol SGD (dynamic display)[8,9]	Line drawings, photos, logos, orthography	High	Dynamic	

*Note. SGD = speech-generating device; many SGDs may also be available as non-dedicated devices
[1] Picture Communication Symbols from BoardMaker: www.mayerjohnson.com   [2] Communication wallet from www.gokeytech.com
[3] Photo taken by the first author
[4] Eye-com board from www.acciinc.com
[5] Big Mack and Little Mack from www.ablenetinc.com   [6] Bluebird II, Go Talk 20 from www.saltillo.com
[7] MessageMate 40 from www.words-plus.com
[8] Vantage Lite from www.prentrom.com
[9] DynaVox V and DynaWrite from www.dynavoxtech.com

17

Table 1-4

Multimodal Communication of a Young Child with Down Syndrome

Communication behavior	Communication mode	Unaided or aided
Vocalizes to gain father's attention	Speech	Unaided
Signs DRINK	Manual sign	Unaided
Points to photo of juice	Gesture	Unaided
Makes face of disgust and sticks out tongue	Facial expression	Unaided
Uses index finder to select "chocolate milk" on computerized voice output device	AAC	Aided (direct selection on high-tech dynamic display device)

You can see, then, that there are many different types of AAC that are available. Later, we'll discuss some of the basics of matching a given person's profile with the types of AAC options that are available. For now, one of the most important points to remember is that nearly all people are *multi-modal communicators*. For example, virtually every person who can use even very simple symbols (such as photographs of food items) and who has some volitional movement of his or her body will use both unaided and aided communication. Look, for example, at the communication behaviors of the young boy with Down syndrome listed in Table 1.4. This boy communicated five different messages using five distinct communication modes. You could use this table format to identify each mode of communication mode and categorize each of your own communication behaviors in the last 24 hours.

When and Where do People Use AAC?

Now that you have an idea of what AAC is and who might use it, we need to think about when it is important for someone to have access to AAC, and in what settings AAC might be used. First, take a moment to make a list of all the ways in which you have communicated with someone, and the ways in which others have communicated with you, within the last 24 hours. Think broadly: include both face-to-face communication and distance communication, and also spoken and written communication. Once you have finished your list, compare it with the examples below, and consider if you missed anything. Here are some of the possibilities:

1. Spoken communication:
   a. Face-to-face communication with: family, friends, classmates, clerks, bus drivers, teachers, colleagues at work, pets
   b. Distance communication (personal): phone, video messaging, Skype™
   c. Distance communication (non-personal): TV shows, YouTube™, DVDs

2. Written communication:
   a. Personal: grocery lists, text messages, emails, letters, notes to/from family/roommates on the kitchen counter/refrigerator/white board, schedule books, PDA, Facebook™
   b. Non-personal: mail, textbooks, novels, magazines, cookbooks, road signs, advertisements, maps, GPS, website surfing

The list could go on and on. You communicate – or are being communicated to – nearly all time, in nearly every conceivable setting; not just when you are talking with your best friend, but also when you are reading a textbook or a website, or watching a movie, or reading exit signs on the freeway. In the latter cases, the sender of the message (i.e., the textbook and website authors, movie directors and actors, and signage designers) may have created messages that the receiver obtains far after their original creation, sometimes even decades later. Note that the ways we communicate can be classified as spoken or written, and that any given moment of communication is primarily receptive or expressive in nature. Table 1.5 includes multiple examples of various spoken and written methods of communication that are either primarily expressive or receptive in nature. Using the list of communication methods in Table 1.5, as well as your own list of how you've communicated in the last day, create and fill out a table using the same headings as 1.5.

Table 1.5

Examples of Various Spoken and Written Communication Methods

	Spoken	Written
Receptive	1. Phone: Listening to your father tell you about his excursion to an antique shop 2. Radio: listening to National Public Radio on your way to school 3. MP3 player: listening to music during your morning run	1. Internet: Reading a blog about the day's national and international news 2. Email: Reading a message from your professor about an assignment 3. Twitter ^{TM}: Reading a tweet from a favorite band
Expressive	1. Phone: Telling your best friend about your date last night 2. Voice text: Leaving a message for a friend about meeting for coffee 3. Face-to-face: Placing your order at the coffee shop	1. Email: Asking a classmate for notes that you are missing 2. Facebook ^{TM}: Posting photos and descriptions of a recent weekend getaway 3. Text message: Texting your sister about babysitting your nieces

In addition to considering various *methods* of communication, we must consider the *purposes* of communication. For example, think about all the reasons why you might send someone a text message: to confirm a time for dinner, to ask someone to pick up an item at the store on the way home, to check on your children, to flirt, or to gossip (possibly even while sitting in class)! Light (1989) identified four main purposes for communicating:

- to engage in social etiquette routines, for example, saying hello to your classmate when you sit down in class
- to gain social closeness, as when we talk with friends and family, or post/read information on Facebook™, or join an electronic dating service
- to gather and/or transfer information, for example, when you research a topic for class on the Internet
- to express needs and wants, as when a child asks a parent for a candy bar at the grocery store

These four communicative purposes – to engage in social etiquette routines, establish and maintain social closeness, transfer information, and express needs and wants – are central to the human experience. The methods by which we communicate with each other have evolved (or, some might say devolved!) over time, particularly with regard to the various forms of electronic communication, but the purposes remain fairly constant.

In many essential ways, the communication needs for people who use AAC may be the same as your communication needs. They are people like you (or like your children, parents, or grandparents) who want and need to communicate in many different ways for a wide variety of purposes. However, individuals who use AAC may have difficulty with any or all of methods of communication listed above, and with the four purposes of communication. Your job as an SLP, then, is to ensure that your AAC clients have access to the fullest possible range of communication modes and purposes, given each person's specific desires, needs, and abilities. The answer to the question, then, of when and where people need to use

AAC, is that people need access to effective means of communication any time and any place where communication takes place. In future chapters, we will examine how to go about assessing an individual's communication needs and abilities, and also some basic principles for providing appropriate intervention and instruction to ensure the person is reaching his or her communication potential. First, however, let us examine various work settings where SLPs may encounter people with AAC needs.

CHAPTER 2

AAC Across Clinical Settings

Now that you have a good idea of what kinds of people might need AAC, let's talk about the settings in which you might work with people who have AAC needs. As you probably know, SLPs work in an extraordinarily wide range of settings, from preschools to nursing homes. Similarly, people with AAC needs can be found within nearly all of the same settings. Let's take a look at some of those settings, starting with settings for young children and working our way through the lifespan.

Early Intervention (Birth to Three) Programs

By federal law, all families in the United States who have very young children with disabilities and who meet set criteria are eligible for birth-to-three services within their natural environments. Typically, for this young population, services are provided within the child's home. SLPs who work with this population, then, typically do a lot of traveling to visit families and children in their homes. For a child to be identified as having a disability at such a young age, this frequently means that the child has a significant disability. Children may, for example, have been born very prematurely. They may have any of a number of congenital syndromes (e.g., Down syndrome, Prader-Willi syndrome), may have experienced trauma during birth (e.g., lack of oxygen resulting from having the umbilical cord wrapped around the neck), or may have experienced some type of extreme trauma after birth (e.g., shaken baby syndrome or other form of traumatic brain injury). Many of these children may benefit from receiving AAC services very early on in life. Remember, typically developing children start understanding words by approximately nine months of age and start speaking by approximately twelve months of age (Owens, 2008) and they have spent all of their months prior to that time absorbing all of the speech and language surrounding them. It is important, then, to ensure access to appropriate means of communication even from the very beginning of life, and to provide AAC services even to these very young children.

Preschools

Preschool children usually range from about three to five years of age. Some preschool settings are private, in which parents pay to enroll their child, and some programs are funded at least in part by the state and/or federal government, with one of the largest of these being the Head Start program. Children who qualify for speech and language services typically can attend a preschool program, and certainly can receive SLP (and other) services, free of charge. A number of preschool children will have speech and/or language impairments that are significant enough to warrant the use of AAC. In fact, recent survey findings indicated that preschool SLPs had an average of seven children with AAC needs on their caseloads (Binger, 2006). Children in this setting may have a wide range of disorders and will, of course, include many of the same children served by birth-to-three services. They may include children who have a primary disability of general developmental delays (some of whom may, later on, be diagnosed with intellectual impairment), autism spectrum disorder, multiple disabilities (possibly resulting from a genetic syndrome), deaf-blind, or any of a number of other disorders. These children may be classified as having a number of secondary disorders as well, such as cerebral palsy, hearing impairment, or visual impairment.

Provision of appropriate AAC solutions is crucial for this population for a number of reasons. So much language development takes place during the first five years of life, and appropriate AAC provision helps to ensure children are achieving their maximum communication potentials. Appropriate AAC solutions will allow preschoolers with disabilities to participate in all of the same activities as their typically developing peers, such as selecting and singing songs during circle time and participating in a wide range of activities like story reading, arts and crafts, learning centers, and free play. In addition, toward the end of the child's preschool years, the AAC team (which will be discussed in the next chapter) will consider various educational options for the child, possibly including enrollment in a special education classroom. Many children who have appropriate AAC services in place can function without difficulties within regular education classrooms, but if these services are not in place, the team may be more reluctant to place the child full-time within a regular education classroom. It is critical to ensure that any child who is placed within a special education classroom is there because they genuinely need that type of educational support, rather than because their teams did not have the appropriate AAC solutions available to allow them to function within a typical classroom setting. Therefore, it becomes clear that providing appropriate AAC services to the birth-to-three and preschool populations helps to ensure that children receive appropriate placements in kindergarten and beyond.

Public Schools

SLPs work with students in kindergarten through twelfth grade. As with SLPs who work in preschools, SLPs who work with the school-age populations certainly work with students with AAC needs. Similar to the findings reported for preschoolers, recent survey results have indicated that school-based SLPs had an average of eight students on their caseloads with AAC needs (Kent-Walsh, 2008). The students' backgrounds, disabilities, and AAC needs will vary widely. Some students who use AAC may primarily be enrolled in the same classes as their typical peers. For example, students with cerebral palsy may spend most or all of their time in regular education classrooms; they may rely on AAC for face-to-face communication, and on both AAC and AT solutions for completing academic work. Such a student will require ongoing SLP support throughout all grades, for assistance with both social and academic communication. Other students – particularly those with intellectual impairments, which may or may not be accompanied by physical impairments – may spend part or most of their time within specialized classroom settings, such as a classroom for children on the autism spectrum or for children with profound intellectual impairments. In nearly all cases, a major role of the SLP is to work with classroom teachers and other support personnel (such as educational assistants/paraprofessionals, occupational therapists [OTs], physical therapists [PTs], etc.) to ensure their students are receiving the educational supports that they need. It should also be noted that children enrolled in private schools may receive school-based SLP services. In most of these cases, an SLP will have a contract with an individual school in order to provide SLP services (including AAC services).

Hospitals

Hospital settings can vary dramatically. Clients with AAC needs in this setting may range across the lifespan, from a child with a traumatic brain injury from a car accident to an elderly adult with a stroke. Some SLPs work in non-specialized hospitals in which patients with an enormous range of impairments are seen, and some work in specialized hospitals, such as a rehabilitation hospital for individuals with traumatic brain injuries. SLPs may work in intensive care, acute care, or rehabilitation settings. They may only see inpatients, only see outpatients, or see a combination of both. Regardless, SLPs in any of these hospital settings are extremely likely to have clients with AAC needs. These clients may have temporary AAC needs – for example, someone may have a tracheotomy after surgery that will be removed after a short period of time, but the person is temporarily unable to talk. Another example would be a client with an acquired disorder that has created a more permanent need for AAC, which is the case for many people who have experienced strokes, traumatic brain injuries, or brain tumors. Some SLPs, particularly those working within metropolitan areas, may run specialty clinics within hospitals that primarily focus on clients who need AAC, such as a clinic for people who have amytrophic lateral sclerosis (ALS, also known as Lou Gehrig's disease). As we discussed in Chapter 1, any of these clients who have communication needs that cannot be met by using their speech can potentially benefit from using AAC.

Nursing Homes/Long-Term Care Facilities

SLPs often work in nursing homes with clients who have some form of dementia, such as Alzheimer's disease. In many cases, SLP services may focus primarily on issues relating to dysphagia (i.e., swallowing disorders), as funding for dysphagia treatment tends to be more available with this population than for other types of treatment. However, evidence suggests that clients certainly can benefit from a wide range of AAC options, such as the use of photo albums/memory books, communication notebooks, wallets, cards, and even some high tech AAC solutions (Beukelman, 2005). Using AAC with this population helps to support the client's memory, and it also can help provide contexts for communication for both the client and for the communication partners (e.g., family, nursing home staff). SLPs also may see clients with other types of disorders within long-term care facilities, including younger as well as older clients with degenerative disorders (such as ALS or multiple sclerosis), and clients with other types of disorders that are so significant that the person can no longer be cared for at home, either temporarily or permanently.

Private Practice

Another setting in which SLPs work and see clients with AAC needs is within private practices. Private practice settings can vary dramatically. One example is an outpatient clinic that is a part of a private hospital system (these may exist for publicly-owned hospitals as well). Services may be provided in a clinic within a main hospital or, in the case of some metropolitan areas, the hospital may have one or more satellite clinics where SLP, OT, and PT therapy services are conducted. Some clinics may focus exclusively on pediatric populations; this clientele may consist of children of all ages whose families are seeking services to supplement the services they receive in school. Other clinics may focus on the adult population; here, the majority of clients are likely to be adults with recently acquired disorders such as strokes and traumatic brain injuries who have been released from the hospital. In addition, many SLPs have their own private practices, and they may work alone or employ a number of other therapists (typically SLPs, OTs, and/or PTs). Depending on the populations they serve, these clinicians may or may not have an actual clinic; instead, they may see clients in their natural environments. For example, SLPs who are contracted to provide services to adults with developmental disorders typically go to their clients' homes (either family homes or group homes, depending on where they live), employment settings, or sheltered workshops to provide services. Adults with developmental disorders, particularly the middle-aged and aging population, have historically been highly underserved with respect to AAC. It is unfortunate that many clients could have benefited tremendously from being provided with AAC services years and even decades earlier, but instead were left with few means of communication. Private practice SLPs in some communities may also be contracted to provide services in any of the other settings previously mentioned including: schools, hospitals, and long-term care facilities. Finally, some SLPs with private practices may choose to specialize in working with the AAC population, thereby becoming a tremendous resource for their communities.

As you can see, then, if you are an SLP, the setting in which you choose to work does not really matter: regardless of your work place, in all likelihood, you will be working with individuals who use AAC. In the next chapter, we will take a closer look at the other key people who are likely to be involved with clients who use AAC.

CHAPTER 3

Key Players in
AAC Service-Delivery

Now that you've looked at many of the different settings in which you might work with people who use AAC, do you have some idea of the other individuals who might be involved in providing services for this population? In this chapter, we will discuss who the key players are likely to be, what roles they might play in the lives of the individuals who use AAC, and which people might be responsible for various components of AAC intervention. First, though, let's examine the roles and responsibilities of the SLP, as stipulated by the American Speech-Language-Hearing Association (ASHA, 2005):

- Recognize and hold paramount the needs and interests of individuals who may benefit from AAC and assist them to communicate in ways they desire.
- Implement a multimodal approach to enhance effective communication that is culturally and linguistically appropriate.
- Acquire and maintain the knowledge and skills that are necessary to provide quality professional services.
- Integrate perspectives, knowledge and skills of team members, especially those individuals who have AAC needs, their families, and significant others in developing functional and meaningful goals and objectives.
- Assess, intervene, and evaluate progress and outcomes associated with AAC interventions using principles of evidence-based practice.
- Facilitate individuals' uses of AAC to promote and maintain their quality of life.
- Advocate with and for individuals who can or already do benefit from AAC, their families, and significant others to address

communication needs and ensure rights to full communication access.

We have already addressed a number of these issues, such as taking a multimodal approach to communication. In this chapter, we will pay particular attention to the fourth item on the list – that is, integrating information from a variety of team members. We will begin with a list of people who might have a significant role to play in the lives of someone using AAC:

- person who uses AAC
- family members/ significant others: spouse/ domestic partner/ boyfriend/ girlfriend, parents, grandparents, children, siblings, other relatives
- SLP
- OT
- PT
- social worker/ case manager
- audiologist and/or vision specialist
- classroom teacher, special education teacher, and/or educational assistant
- school psychologist and/or behavior therapist
- nurse, physician, and/or surgeon
- Respiratory therapist, and/or nutritionist
- aides and staff (nursing homes, group homes, sheltered workshops)
- friends/ peers/ neighbors

That is quite a list, right? Of course, no one person who uses AAC will be involved with everyone on the list, but many people who use AAC – particularly those with fragile medical conditions – may have a large number of professionals involved in their lives, in addition to their family and friends. If the person is very young, very old, or simply unable to leave home frequently, a family literally may have over a dozen professionals in and out of their home on an ongoing basis. Alternatively, a family may spend a great deal of time transporting someone who uses

AAC from one appointment to the next. Let's take a look at the responsibilities of these various people.

Roles of AAC Team Members

First, it has been argued that the person using AAC should have as much say as possible over decisions in his or her life (Glennen, 1997), which includes, whenever possible, decisions regarding AAC. Family members also have a significant stake in AAC choices; if family members do not "buy into" AAC decisions, they are unlikely to follow the recommendations. For example, if the SLP recommends a complex, high tech AAC device for an elderly man with an acquired disorder (such as a stroke), and neither the man nor his wife have any experience with technology and are extremely reluctant to touch the device, let alone use it for communication, it is highly unlikely that the intervention will be successful.

The SLP's role, then, is not simply to independently conduct an AAC assessment and come up with recommendations based on the client's communication profile (which we will discuss in the next chapter). It is true that the SLP is the person who is primarily responsible for planning and conducting AAC assessments and interventions, but this role must be a collaborative one in order to achieve success. The SLP must work as a team with the individual who uses AAC, the family, and a range of professionals to make joint decisions, if true success is to be attained – that is, finding and implementing AAC solutions that meet both the short-term and long-term needs of the client.

In the remainder of this chapter, we will examine the roles of: (a) AAC team members, such as OTs, PTs, and social workers/case managers, who work across a wide range of settings, much like SLPs (Glennen, 1997), and (b) other team members, such as educators and physicians) who are involved in only specific service-delivery settings.

Generally speaking, OTs focus on ensuring maximal function in everyday life, including everything from being able to get dressed in the morning to performing job-related activities. They may focus on fine motor impairments (such as fine motor control of the hands) and also sensory integration impairments (that is, integrating input from all of our senses – tactile, visual, etc.; impairments in this area are common among children with communication disorders). PTs generally focus more on gross motor impairments, such as working to improve someone's ability to walk. However, there is much overlap between these two professions. If the person using AAC has significant motor impairments, then the OT and/or PT may play a critical role on the AAC team. These professionals will work collaboratively with the SLP to determine how the person will access aided AAC solutions. For example, some individuals with cerebral palsy may need to use switches to access their devices, instead of using their index fingers or hands. Switches can be accessed by reliable motor movements nearly anywhere on the body, such as the head, elbow, knee, foot, or even eyebrow. The OT /PT ensures that the client is properly positioned, has maximal use of all residual movement, and is using AAC access methods that will not cause any further physical challenges (for example, to ensure the movement used to access a switch does not trigger a motor reflex pattern).

Social workers, who also sometimes function as case managers and oversee the details of a client's case, can be found in all of the settings discussed in Chapter 2. A social worker in a Head Start program may, for example, ensure that the child's family has access to a range of government programs, such as programs that assist with the provision of food and shelter, as well as other programs that are specifically designed for families with disabilities (e.g., provide funding assistance for therapies and specialized child care and medical needs).

Professionals who specialize in sensory impairments will be consulted as the need arises. It is quite common for people who use AAC to have hearing and/or vision impairments, so when the need arises, the SLP or other professionals will refer clients to audiologists and vision specialists for testing. These professionals may be consulted on an as-needed basis for helping with AAC decision-making. For example, a vision specialist might help determine how sharp the color contrasts need to be on an AAC display for the client to see them clearly.

Other professionals on AAC teams will only be found within particular settings. In school settings (preschool, primary, and secondary), the student's educators will be involved, particularly the classroom teacher, special education teacher, and educational assistant. Educators play critical roles on AAC teams. They are the people who spend the most time with students in the school environment and they have a primary role in ensuring maximal exposure to age- and developmentally-appropriate curricula. The SLP must work hand-in-hand with the educational staff to ensure that AAC solutions help meet the student's educational goals. For example, the SLP will work closely with educators to ensure that a student has access to vocabulary that is needed for a particular academic unit, such as vocabulary relating to sea life and ocean currents if the class is completing a unit on oceans. Other school support staff may include school psychologists, who are typically responsible for psychological and intellectual testing, and behavior specialists, who are involved with students who exhibit challenging behaviors. It is critical for the SLP to work closely with these professionals with many students who use AAC, as challenging behaviors frequently result from the student lacking effective means of communication (Downing, 2005). It should also be noted that some school districts or special education units have assistive technology teams in place; these teams typically provide supports for AAC as well as other AT needs. The people on this team may or may not work full-time on the AT team, depending on the size of the district. SLPs, OTs, PTs, and special educators all may serve on the AT team. Frequently, the AT team is called in to consult with a student's immediate AAC team (i.e., primary SLP, classroom educators, educational assistants, etc.). The AT team typically will conduct an initial AAC assessment, make AAC recommendations, and provide follow-up services for the student's AAC team.

A different set of professionals will be involved with clients or patients who are in medical settings, such as hospitals and nursing homes. Nurses, physicians, surgeons, respiratory therapists, nutritionists, and various aides may all be involved with clients in these settings. The extent of their roles on AAC teams will vary, depending on the setting and client. Professionals on an Intensive Care Unit in a hospital may only work with a patient for a very short period of time, compared with nursing home staff, who may be involved with their clients for much longer periods. In the former case, the amount of time an SLP spends working with the staff to promote AAC is often relatively limited for any given patient, whereas an SLP may work together with the staff in a long-term care facility (or in a group home or sheltered workshop) over a longer period of time to come up with AAC solutions that will work in both the short- and long-term for both the client and the staff.

Finally, we must not neglect the role that friends and peers may play on an AAC team. Their roles will vary, depending on their closeness to the client or student and on their willingness and availability for participation. Close friends can provide valuable information when devising AAC systems – for example, they can provide critical information that can help with vocabulary selection for AAC systems that even a family member might not know. For example, if a retired man with a stroke wants to return to his weekly coffee shop visit with his male friends, only those friends will be able to provide information as to the specifics of common topics of conversation. Friends and/or peers also may play an important role in intervention. A student at school, for example, may benefit from having a "peer buddy," who has received some instruction from the SLP, and who can help show the student using AAC how to communicate more effectively by using the device within various school activities (Binger, 2008).

You can see, then, that many different people can play critical roles when providing services to individuals who use AAC. Some of these people may assist primarily with the AAC assessment process, some with intervention, and some with many different aspects of service delivery. Now that you have an idea of the types of people who might need AAC, some of the work settings in which you will find those clients, and some of the key people who will be involved, we will take a closer look at how to complete the process of assessing the exact AAC needs of clients who need AAC.

CHAPTER 4

AAC Assessment Basics

Although we cannot go into the details of how to do an AAC assessment in this book, we can give you an overview of what AAC assessments are all about and discuss some of the basic principles that apply to completing AAC assessments. As you probably know, SLP assessments are usually conducted to determine if the client has a disorder or not, and to carefully describe, and sometimes diagnose, the disorder if it exists. When SLPs conduct an AAC assessment, it usually is very clear to everyone that the client has some type of disorder, and in all likelihood, the client has had at least one, if not numerous, prior SLP evaluations. Some of the goals, then, of conducting an AAC assessment are somewhat different from the goals of other SLP assessments. Although it is important to develop a communication profile and gain an understanding of the client's communication challenges, with an AAC assessment, the primary focus is not on diagnosing a disorder. Instead, the focus is on considering, with each AAC assessment task, how the client might use AAC to enhance his daily life communication. In an AAC assessment, we systematically search for the client's strengths, with a very practical focus on how those strengths can be used to help the person communicate (see Principles 6 and 7).

That is not to say that we will not assess many of the same areas that we assess in more traditional speech and language evaluations. We may, for example, systematically assess the following areas during an AAC assessment (Beukelman, 2005): natural speech, motor ability (seating, positioning, fine motor abilities), cognition, symbol comprehension and expression (including the symbol types discussed in Chapter 1), language comprehension and expression (semantics, syntax, morphology), pragmatics, literacy, and sensory/ perceptual (vision, hearing). At times, we may use techniques that differ from more traditional speech and language evaluations; for example, if a client has severe motor limitations, instead of having the client choose from multiple pictures on a page of a language comprehension test by pointing to the chosen item (e.g., pointing to a picture indicating "run" following the prompt, "Show me run"), we may use partner-assisted scanning instead, in which the partner points to one picture on a page at a time while asking, "Is it this one?," with the client indicating "yes" or "no" via head nod/shake, thumbs up/down, or some other method. However, the description of the client's skills on tasks such as standardized tests is not necessarily very different from those within other assessments. What does differ is how we view and use that information. The information that we gather is used, very directly, to make AAC decisions. For example, if clients have literacy skills that are intact, then we will explore using AAC devices that are orthographically based. If children are able to comprehend simple sentence structures, then we will ensure they also have communication modes available for producing simple sentences, so we can support their ongoing communication development.

AAC assessments differ in additional ways from more traditional SLP assessments, as discussed in the remainder of this chapter. The below ten principles have been adapted from an AAC textbook (Lloyd, 1997) and are intended to give you a sense of the goals, priorities, and the scope of conducting AAC assessments.

Principle 1: Everyone Can and Does Communicate

It has been said that one cannot *not* communicate. We communicate all the time, even when we do not intend to do so. Have you, for example, ever glanced at your watch while talking with a friend or sitting in class? Whether you meant to or not, you communicated that you are thinking about transitioning into another activity (or that you are bored, or late, etc). As we discussed earlier, communication can take various forms – it is not just about talking. Even people with the most profound disabilities communicate in some way – with their gaze, by smiling, or by using any of a number of other ways to communicate. AAC assessments are based on this premise, and one of the aims of conducting an AAC assessment is to document the client's current methods of communication.

Principle 2: AAC Assessments Must be Consumer Responsive

The term "consumers" can be applied to people in many situations, and it is helpful here in illustrating that clients and students – and their families – have a large stake in the outcomes of clinical decisions. As we discussed in Chapter 3, we must include and carefully consider the needs of our clients and their families if our decisions are to create meaningful, positive change. When possible, we should encourage clients to take charge of their own service delivery needs (Blackstone, 1994), as they are the people most affected by decisions that are made.

Principle 3: AAC Assessments Must be Conducted by Collaborative Teams

As we discussed in Chapter 3, many people may be included on a person's AAC team. In order for an AAC assessment to lead to functional outcomes for the client, it is essential that AAC teams function collaboratively. This sounds easier than it is – different people on the team may have a different view as to what is best for the client. Teams must agree on critical issues such as who has authority on the team, of what that authority consists, and the roles and responsibilities for each team member (Giangreco, 1990). For example, imagine that an SLP decides that an educational assistant (EA) will do much of the programming on a student's AAC device and recommends a device based on this assumption. However, the EA and classroom teacher were not involved in this decision. The EA may feel resentful that such a decision was made without his involvement. Further, he may be reluctant to take on this task due to a lack of comfort and experience with technology. In addition, the classroom teacher is upset because she is worried about how much time the EA will have to devote to programming, when the EA is also needed for much hands-on work with the students in the class. You can see how a well-intentioned decision quickly unravels when decisions are not made collaboratively. In contrast, when teams work closely and collaboratively, they can achieve very positive outcomes, with every team member feeling that he or she has a stake in the client's success and a way to help achieve such success (Soto, 2001).

Principle 4: AAC Assessment Must Focus on Functional, Daily Life Activities

SLP students receive much instruction on conducting assessments within clinical settings. A typical assessment session for someone with a communication disorder typically involves conducting interviews and gathering case information from the client and family, performing a hearing screening, administering a battery of standardized tests, and completing informal observations in the clinic. Although this approach may be fine for many individuals – for example, a child who has an articulation disorder – it will not suffice for individuals who use AAC. Helping a person who uses AAC to maximize his or her participation in everyday life is a major focus of AAC intervention; therefore, the team must focus the AAC assessment on gathering information which will lead to AAC solutions that will affect daily life. For example, the SLP may complete a series of classroom observations not only with the student who is being assessed but also with a same-age, same-gender peer, with a goal of identifying participation gaps (Beukelman, 2005). In many cases, AAC may be used to help bridge those gaps. Similar information must be collected for adults who are being assessed. For example, as we mentioned earlier, critical information regarding relevant topics of conversation may be gained from collecting information from the friends with whom a man has coffee once a week. This is the type of information that can make or break AAC interventions; unless the focus is on improving functional outcomes, it is unlikely that AAC solutions will yield positive results.

Principle 5: Focus on Functional Implications of the Disorder, not the Disorder Itself

This principle is closely related to Principle 4, as it also focuses on functional outcomes, and contrasts AAC assessments with other SLP assessments. Often an initial assessment with a client who has a communication disorder focuses extensively on diagnosing and describing the disorder(s) that the client has – for example, test results and observations that lead to the diagnosis of apraxia of speech, aphasia, specific language impairment, etc. Such an approach is both required and useful for many assessments – for example, accurate diagnoses provide guidance toward appropriate intervention techniques and can assist with ensuring clients will qualify for SLP services. However, AAC assessments do not focus on the disability or pathology itself. AAC assessment is not about describing what the client can't do; instead, it must focus, in part, on the *impact* the disability has on functional daily life. For example, a person with aphasia can be described in terms of the disability's negative impact on language functions, such as the ability to form complete sentences, retrieve words accurately, and comprehend spoken and written language. This information is useful for diagnosing aphasia, but it does not lead us directly to appropriate, functional AAC solutions. However, if we gather information on how these difficulties impact the client's daily life – for example, that he has difficulty answering questions about daily life events, such as where he is going with his wife tonight – then we have a better idea of some of the types of AAC solutions we might try. In this case, one possibility would be to provide the client with written choices to assist comprehension; for example, the SLP asks, "Where are you going with your wife tonight: To the movies, out to a restaurant, or to your children's house?" while writing the words *movie, restaurant,* and *children*, to see if the client can make the correct selection (Beukelman, 2005).

Principle 6: Focus on Strengths and Abilities

Placing a focus on the client's strengths in an AAC assessment is not about being politically correct; it is an absolute fundamental and highly practical approach to assessment. By way of example, we can consider a child with severe cerebral palsy. We quickly see that she uses a wheelchair, has little voluntary movement of her legs, has little use of her left arm or hand, and her speech is highly unintelligible. If we perform an assessment and share this information with her family, we fall into two traps: we have become yet another set of professionals who are (a) telling them what they already know, and (b) telling them what is wrong with their daughter. Instead, by focusing on her strengths, we find that she is

40

able to use her right index finger to point to fairly small targets – which means she likely will able to direct select on an AAC device. We also discover in our assessment that she can identify a wide array of concepts (nouns, verbs, adjectives, etc.) that are depicted by photographs and line drawings, which tells us that she may be able to use these types of symbols to communicate. Therefore, instead of telling her parents what is wrong with her (yet again), we can begin to discuss functional modes of communication that will support her development. Certainly, we must take note of what our clients are not able to do – perhaps, for example, this child cannot yet combine symbols or use a computerized display – but we must find out what they *can* do in order to identify appropriate AAC solutions that will be functional for our clients.

Principle 7: Focus on Feature Matching

Feature matching means that the skills of the client are matched to the features of an AAC system (Glennen, 1997). In our previous example, the child with cerebral palsy has the ability to point with her index finger, which can then be matched up with the feature of using direct selection to access aided AAC. She also has the ability to identify a variety of photos and line drawings, so we will match this skill with devices in which she can use those types of symbols. In the example of the man with aphasia, he has the ability to make selections from a range of written choices, so we can match that skill the use of the written choice communication technique. If a client had functional literacy skills, we would ensure that any aided AAC options would make use of this skill. Alternatively, if a child has a significant intellectual impairment and cannot yet identify photographs, but he can communicate by pointing to what he wants and using other unaided means of communication (tugging on people, facial expressions), we may place a primary focus on working to expand his unaided communication means to ensure that he has a function means of communication, while also introducing more symbolic means of communication as appropriate. Thus, a major part of AAC assessment is to use the information that we gain pertaining to the client's skills and abilities and apply it to specific AAC solutions.

Principle 8: Adhere to the Law of Parsimony

The law of parsimony, otherwise known as "Occam's razor," states that "entities should not be multiplied unnecessarily." Or, to put it another way, "the simplest explanation for a phenomenon is most likely the correct explanation." When we apply this principle to AAC assessments, it means that we must do our best, in the midst of so many different and sometimes competing perspectives and factors (person using AAC, family members, other AAC team members, other communication partners, various environments, multi-component AAC systems), to keep this inherently complex process as simple as possible. Conducting an AAC assessment may be complicated, but it should not become so overwhelming that it takes an unreasonable amount of time to complete and results in more questions than answers. Similarly, we should do our best to ensure that we are providing our clients with AAC solutions that meet their communication needs using the simplest solutions possible. This axiom relates to the next principle in that no AAC assessment will answer all questions; it is enough, sometimes, to have enough of a start to assist the client in identifying a path toward more functional communication.

Principle 9: Assessment is an Ongoing Process

Life is change: that adage is just as true for people who use AAC as for anyone else. Add to that the fact that we frequently cannot learn everything we need to know in an initial assessment, and it is easy to see why AAC assessment is an ongoing process. In some cases, conducting follow-up assessment tasks may be fairly predictable. For example, if a student is transitioning from high school into a work place, we know ahead of time that this transition will be taking place; in fact, schools are required to begin planning for such transitions years in advance. Another example is people who have degenerative disorders, such as ALS or dementia. We do not necessarily know how rapidly their level of function will change, but we do know that it will, and this allows us to anticipate when further AAC assessment is warranted. In other cases, unanticipated changes may occur that create the need to reassess AAC solutions. For example, someone with ALS may take a rapid turn for the worse.

Alternatively, someone with a traumatic brain injury may regain much more functioning than originally expected, such as a soldier returning home with a gunshot wound to the head who has no consistent yes/no response who, within the span of six months, recovers nearly all of his literacy skills – and can therefore use an AAC device that uses orthography, an option that was well beyond his reach at the time of the initial assessment.

Principle 10: AAC Assessment Should Result in Positive Change

Simply put, if we have not made life better for our clients in some tangible way, then we have not done our job adequately. We must collect data on our clients' performance and document changes, and we must revise our plans as needed to ensure ongoing progress.

There, then, are some general principles that apply to virtually all AAC assessments. Hopefully, these principles leave you with a strong sense that AAC assessment is focused on functional, daily life communication, and also that AAC assessment is about much more than about finding the "right" piece of technology for someone. AAC, after all, is simply a tool; if we fail to consider how that tool will be used within a broader context, it will very likely be found collecting dust in a cabinet.

CHAPTER 5

AAC Intervention Basics

In the last chapter, we stressed the differences between AAC assessments and typical speech and language assessments, particularly with respect to AAC assessments focusing on the client strengths and capabilities for using AAC systems, instead of on speech and language deficits. Here, however, we will take somewhat of an opposite approach by stressing the fact that AAC interventions should not be so different from other speech and language interventions that they seem completely foreign. Like interventions for people with communication disorders who are mainly relying on speech to communicate, the SLP is the primary person on the team who is responsible for communication interventions for people who cannot rely on natural speech to meet all of their communication needs. Similarly, as is the case with any service-delivery team, the only way for AAC interventions to be successful is for the SLP to collaborate with other key players. For example, SLPs commonly collaborate closely with classroom teachers to ensure that children with language disorders receive the support they need in classroom situations; similar collaboration also is essential to promote successful communication outcomes for children who use AAC. With adults, the focus is commonly placed on helping family members learn to facilitate communication with the person who has a communication disorder, whether AAC is used or not. Therefore, in every case, child or adult, the focus of intervention is on creating improvements in the daily life functioning of the client, not in promoting isolated skills in the therapy room. Thus, in most or all cases, the SLP is primarily responsible for creating intervention plans based on AAC assessment findings, but the whole AAC team typically needs to be involved in the implementation of those plans.

Best Practices for AAC Instruction

Throughout this book, we have stressed the importance of focusing on functional, real life outcomes for people who use AAC; there is little point to providing AAC services if those services do not result in an improved quality of life for our clients or their loved ones. There are certain steps we can take throughout the process of providing services to this population to help ensure this outcome (Glennen & DeCoste, 1997):

1. We should ensure that our interventions are age-appropriate. For example, if you are working with an adult client who has an intellectual impairment and has limited literacy skills, do not use children's books or other child-like materials; instead, use age-appropriate materials containing supportive graphics, such as magazines on topics that are of interest to the client.

2. As much as possible, instruct the individual within natural settings. Typically, this is readily achievable within school or nursing home settings, but it can be challenging within clinical settings such as private practice offices or hospitals. One way to maximize the chances of generalization is to conduct role plays with the client; even some clients with significant cognitive impairments can learn new skills within role plays and generalize the use of those skills to natural settings (Light, 1998). For example, an adult with autism may use role plays to help him learn to use an introductory strategy on his SGD when he meets new people. This strategy might include the use of a message such as "Hi, I use this computer to talk to people. If you don't understand what I say, you can read the screen or ask me to repeat myself." He can practice using the strategy within role plays with the SLP (who pretends to be someone such as a clerk or a waitress) and then try it out in natural settings.

3. Communication should be taught as an embedded skill. For example, the young man with autism, previously discussed, who is using an introductory strategy needs to practice using this skill within the context of what really would happen when

he meets someone new. Instead of just telling him, "Use this when you meet someone new," we need to have him practice using this skill with all of the cues and responses that happen in the real world (Light, 1998). For example, in role plays, the waitress (played by the SLP) might say, "Hi, my name is Rachel, what can I get you?" during one interaction, and then she might ignore the client entirely the next time and instead ask his friend, "What does he want to eat?" If we do not teach our clients to use their communication skills as they are embedded within natural environments, we should not be surprised when they fail to make progress.

4. An essential part of AAC intervention, as we have alluded to earlier in this book, is working not only with our AAC clients but also with their communication partners. Research has shown that communication partners often do not naturally provide supportive opportunities for individuals using AAC to communicate; partners tend to dominate interactions, predominantly ask yes/no questions, take the majority of conversational turns, and frequently interrupt the communicative attempts of individuals using AAC (Kent-Walsh & McNaughton, 2005). Although these findings may seem discouraging, research also has very clearly indicated that it is possible to create dramatic improvements in the communication of clients who use AAC when we work with their communication partners, even if we do not work directly with the person using AAC (Binger, 2008; Rosa-Lugo & Kent-Walsh, 2008). For example, by teaching parents and educators of children who use AAC how to use techniques such as modeling use of the AAC device and providing the child with plenty of time to communicate, we see increases in the child's use of AAC. Similarly, we may teach the spouse of a person with aphasia to help their loved one to understand and express himself better by the partner supplementing their own speech with visual aids, such as writing down choices (e.g., "What's

your preference for vacation this year: *Alaska, Hawaii,* or *Spain*?" while writing down each choice).

5. As discussed in Chapter 3, working with clients who have AAC needs is a team effort. To be effective, AAC teams must work collaboratively. This may sound simple, but in reality, it can be extremely challenging. What would you do as the SLP, for example, if your assessment results indicated that your client would benefit the most from a particular SGD, but the family of the client is much more interested in a different SGD that you think is inappropriate for the client? Or what would you do if a new student who has an SGD moves into your district and you are the only person on the team who is not defensive about learning to use the SGD? These types of conflicts are very common, and working to resolve them has little to do with being 'nice.' Instead, the issue is ensuring successful outcomes with our clients. If we do not do the hard work of successful collaboration, our clients are the ones who suffer.

6. Finally, on a related note, we must take an integrated approach to the AAC services we provide. In school settings, this means integrating AAC within classroom settings and within student curricula (Zangari, 2009). In other settings, this typically means integrating AAC within whatever functional daily life activities are important to the client, whether that means integrating services within a nursing home, providing a child with a way to tell their mother what they want in a department store, or ensuring that a client can communicate with members of their synagogue, bowling league, or veterans' group.

Communicative Competence

Now that you have an idea of some of the basic principles for providing AAC interventions, let us examine a framework that frequently is used to ensure that clinicians are targeting all key areas of communication for their clients. When a person exhibits communicative competence, they have the knowledge and skills to communicate functionally and can adequately meet their daily communication needs (Light, 1989). There are four major areas of communicative competence, each of which is discussed below: linguistic, operational, social, and strategic. When we set goals and implement intervention with our clients who use AAC, we must be sure to provide our clients with ways to achieve competency within all four of these areas.

Linguistic Competence

As we discussed in Chapter 1, a wide variety of factors, such as the type and extent of the disability, can affect a person's ability to communicate – including their ability to learn and use language successfully. This, of course, is true for people with communication disorders whether or not they require AAC. For both populations (that is, those who do and do not need AAC), a major focus of intervention for many clients is building linguistic competence. Linguistic competence, for anyone, involves possessing receptive and expressive competence with the language that you speak, which for most people is the same language that is typically spoken around you. In the U.S., depending on the community in which you live, this might involve learning English, Spanish, a combination of the two, or any of a number of other languages. This is true for someone who uses AAC, as well. For example, a person who uses AAC may live in a bilingual community and have the need to learn both English and Spanish. In addition, however, the person using AAC must also learn the linguistic codes of the AAC solutions they are using, such as line drawings, manual signs, and other codes. It is perhaps not surprising, then, that attaining (or regaining) linguistic competence can pose particular challenges for a person who uses AAC (Blockberger, 2003).

Social Competence

Just as linguistic competence is frequently an issue for people who have communication disorders, social competence often is a common problem as well. Social competence refers to two main areas of communication: (1) sociolinguistic aspects (or pragmatics), which include discourse strategies such as initiating, maintaining, and terminating conversations, interaction functions such as expressing needs and wants, and specific communicative functions such as requesting and protesting; and (2) sociorelational aspects, which include relational skills such as having a positive self image, showing an interest in others and in communication, and putting communication partners at ease (Light, 1989). Individuals who use AAC may demonstrate weaknesses in any of these areas, and therefore may benefit from intervention to address these issues. For example, building social competence is frequently a major focus of intervention for people with autism spectrum disorders, as social impairment is a major part of this particular disorder. Often, people who use AAC require particular social competencies that other people do not need. For example, it may be important for someone who uses AAC to put other people at ease, as many people may not be comfortable when interacting with a person who uses AAC for the first time (Light, 1998).

Strategic Competence

Strategic competence refers to knowing how to compensate for communication losses by using a range of strategies. People with all types of communication disorders use compensatory strategies to compensate for their disabilities. For example, a child with an articulation disorder who cannot say the word "five" intelligibly may hold up five fingers to convey her meaning. With clients who use AAC, strategic competence may include clarifying messages, optimizing communication efficiency and speed, and coping with communication breakdowns. For example, a person with severe dysarthria (slurred speech), which commonly results from having a stroke, may first try to use their speech when conveying a message. If their partner does not understand them, they may repair the breakdown by typing out a message on their SGD or on a low tech alphabet board. A person with aphasia who has severe word finding problems (anomia) may try to tell a waiter what they would like to order but be unable to come up with the word. Several viable ways to repair this breakdown would be locating the appropriate symbols on the SGD or communication wallet, or to point to the photo or written words for what the person wants on the menu. For many people who use aided AAC, compensatory messages can be added to a communication device, such as,

"I have something to say," "I'm starting over," "Take a guess," "Please repeat each word I say," or even, "Forget it." Having quick access to such messages can prevent breakdowns from occurring or can at least help maintain the flow of conversation.

Operational Competence

This competency refers to the technical skills that are required for communication. Of the four competencies discussed, operational competence is the only one that is fairly unique to individuals who use AAC, with certain exceptions, such as a person with a hearing loss who must learn to operate hearing aids. For people who use AAC, operational competence may refer to skills needed for unaided AAC, such as forming the correct hand shapes and movements for manual signs, or for aided AAC, such as operating an SGD. A wide range of skills may be required for aided AAC use, ranging from turning an SGD device on and off, to locating symbols within a communication book or device, to learning how to use a complicated scanning feature. It is important to note that many types of operations require not only motor skills but also cognitive skills. For example, if a person is using an extensive communication book or a high tech SGD and wants to create a message containing multiple concepts, such as *I WENT SHOPPING WITH AUNT GERTRUDE TODAY*, the person not only needs the physical capability to turn the pages of the communication book or select the right buttons on the SGD; she must also remember where each symbol is located and hold the entire message in her memory while searching for each symbol.

Specific Areas to Address During Intervention

By now, you should have a good idea of some principles for providing AAC intervention and the overarching types of competencies that a person who uses AAC needs in order to achieve communicative competence. Finally, let us take a look at just a few of the specific areas that we would commonly work on with someone who uses AAC. While you are reading each section, consider which of the four competencies – linguistic, social, strategic, and operational – might apply to that area.

Individualizing the AAC System

Each person's AAC system must be individualized, whether the system consists of a set of gestures and/or manual signs, a set of graphic symbols (line drawings, photos) on a communication board, an expensive SGD, or any combination of AAC solutions. Each person has unique communication needs, and AAC teams must provide interventions that maximize the functionality of each person's communication system. This may mean ensuring that a very young child has access to symbols that represent favorite foods, toys, and people, an elderly adult has photographs from her past included in her memory book, or an adult with ALS has software that will 'learn' commonly used words so that these words will be predicted more readily when he types his messages.

Selecting Vocabulary

For many people, part of individualizing AAC systems includes selecting vocabulary and then, if the person is using aided AAC, organizing that vocabulary within AAC devices. It should be noted that SLPs do not always have to select vocabulary for everyone who uses AAC. People who are fully literate can use their literacy skills to formulate their own messages, and they may rely on alphabet boards and/or use software on an SGD that allows them to formulate vocabulary as they type. Even for these clients, however, it may be useful to ensure quick, easy access to certain pre-programmed words and phrases, including frequently used messages (e.g., "Hi, how are you today?"), less frequent but urgent messages ("I do not think my respirator is working – please check it immediately"), and a word bank of frequently used words (e.g., see the second example on Table 5.1). For people who are not literate, the AAC team will have to select the vocabulary to which the person has access, which may include selecting vocabulary from scratch as well as using vocabulary pages and programs that have been pre-programmed by SGD manufacturers or posted online by individuals (e.g., www.adaptedlearning.com).

Consider, for a moment, the importance of vocabulary selection. Think about what it would be like to have someone else select all of the words that you can say for the next 24 hours; if the person forgot to provide you with things you'd like to say – a joke or story you'd like to tell, an answer to a question, information you need to share about your health – you are out of luck. Now expand that, and think what it would be like to have that be the case for the next week, month, year, or the rest of your life. It's a frightening prospect, is it not? However, that is precisely the task that is before an SLP who is designing an AAC system for someone else.

You might ask how SLPs go about this daunting task. Usually, an SLP will use a multi-pronged approach to vocabulary selection. There are many ways to collect vocabulary, including the following: observing the client's natural environments and writing down what people say within those environments (which is called an environmental inventory), using published lists of vocabulary words that people use with high frequency (such as those found at http://aac.unl.edu), examining instructional materials in the classroom, interviewing informants about the interests and activities in which the client is involved, asking informants (e.g., spouses, teachers) to keep a diary of words they think clients might need, and modeling language on the AAC device (which is a great way to find out what vocabulary is missing from the device).

Table 5-1

Examples of Options for Organizing Vocabulary

	Examples
Single symbols: One concept per symbol Graphic symbols[1]	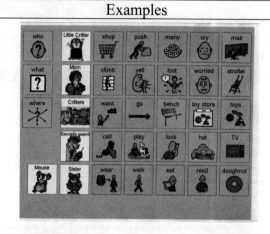
Traditional orthography + line drawings[2]	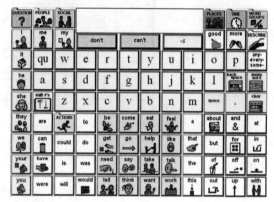

Traditional orthography[3]

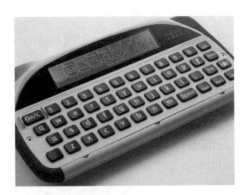

Single symbols: Phrase or sentence[4]

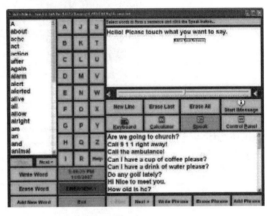

Visual scene: line drawing and photograph[5]

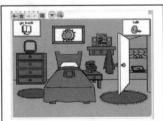

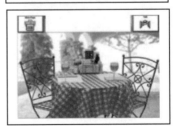

[1] http://www.cathybinger.com/clinical_resources.html
[2] http://www.dynavoxtech.com/gfx/products/wordpower2-lg.gif
[3] http://www.tobiiati.com
[4] http://www.touchntalk.com.
[5] http://www.dynavoxtech.com/products/interaact

Organizing Communication Boards

Once the SLP has collected this information, he or she must decide how to best organize the vocabulary for the client. As discussed in Chapter 1, there is a wide array of "containers" in which AAC symbols can be organized (see Table 1.3), from individual symbols to communication wallets to complex arrays on dynamic display SGDs. Within any type of display, vocabulary may be represented as whole phrases or sentences (as in the respirator example above) or as single concepts (e.g., *I, AM, PLAY*) so that clients can build their own sentences. Single concepts are frequently organized in a *Fitzgerald key* – that is, following the linguistic order of a typical sentence. For an example, see the first figure in Table 5.1, which was designed to go with the Mercer Mayer "Little Critter" book, *Just Shopping with Mom*. In English, this means that subjects are on the left (e.g., Little Critter, Mom,), verbs are toward the center (e.g. shop, climb), and objects toward the right (e.g., mall, stroller). In this way, the person moves from left to right – just as we read from left to right – to build a sentence (*LITTLE CRITTER + SHOP + MALL*). Symbols also can be represented within visual scenes – for example, a person with aphasia may benefit from having photos of himself and his wife in Hawaii available to facilitate talking about a recent vacation (AAC-RERC, 2009), or a very young, contextually-dependent child may benefit from having foods displayed within line drawings or photographs of the kitchen cupboards and refrigerator. See examples of these different ways to organize symbols on Table 5.1.

Facilitating Language Development

Many children and adolescents who use AAC are in the process of developing their receptive and expressive language skills. For these clients, the goals of intervention may not be very different from the goals of clients who are primarily using speech to communicate. Remember, using AAC is not an outcome in and of itself; rather, AAC solutions are simply tools that are used for the greater purpose of communicating – and more specifically, in this case, for developing language skills. For example, both a child who is using AAC and a child who is not may be working toward creating brief sentences that contain a subject, verb, and object, such as the *LITTLE CRITTER + SHOP + MALL* example above. In the first case, the child will be using AAC to create sentences; in the latter case, the child is using speech. In either case, the goal of intervention is the same: to help the child improve syntax skills. The only difference for some clients, then, is that the communication tool changes.

Focusing on Natural Speech

The majority of people who use AAC have at least some use of their voices, and many can form words that are at least partially intelligible. If a person has a choice to communicate by using speech versus using AAC, the person will choose speech, practically every single time. This seems obvious when one considers that speech is efficient, it is always with us, we can say whatever we want, and it is how the vast majority of people talk to each other. For many clients, then, SLP intervention is two-pronged, with a focus on: (1) developing or regaining speech, and (2) maximizing use of AAC solutions. Commonly, families are concerned that using AAC might somehow prevent the development or re-attainment of speech and may therefore be reluctant to introduce AAC. However, a growing body of literature clearly indicates that using AAC does not hinder speech development and may actually help (Millar, 2006; Yoder, 2006; Binger, 2008).

It should be noted that it is not always appropriate to take a two-pronged approach, however. For example, one of the authors once worked with a 22 year old woman with autism who had been receiving SLP services for 20 years. She used very little speech, mainly vowels, and spoke a total of approximately 10 words that her immediate family could understand. Despite this fact, the SLPs who had worked with this client over the years continued to set speech goals for her, such as saying the /p/ and /b/ sounds. Her files reflected that some of these speech goals had been in place for nearly two decades. Clearly, this young woman was not making progress toward functional speech. For this client, then, focusing solely on AAC was a much more appropriate use of everyone's time than continuing to focus on speech development.

Wrap-Up

It is our sincere hope that this book has piqued your interest in the area of AAC and provided you with an overview of the nature of AAC and related clinical issues. As clinicians and researchers who have spent years concentrating on the practice and study of AAC, we can confidently say that AAC is never boring! The variety and breadth of relevant issues allow for infinite opportunities to exercise both creativity and problem-solving skills. Additionally, the ongoing evolution of technologies allows us to keep moving forward with new options to maximize our clients' functional communication. Most importantly, the clients and families with whom we have been privileged to work truly have driven and informed our research and clinical experiences, and these individuals continue to illustrate for us why this area is such a passionate one for us. We are confident that you will have similar experiences and that you will greatly appreciate the work you do relating to AAC!

References

AAC-RERC. (2009, May). AAC for aphasia: A review of visual scenes display project. Retrieved from http://aac-rerc.psu.edu/index-13327.php.html.

American Speech-Language-Hearing Association. (2005). Roles and responsibilities of speech-language pathologists with respect to augmentative communication: Position statement. Retrieved from http://www.asha.org/docs/html/PS2005-00113.html.

Beukelman, D., & Mirenda, P. (2005). *Augmentative and alternative communication: Supporting children and adults with complex communication needs* (3 ed.). Baltimore: Paul H. Brookes Publishing Co.

Binger, C., Berens, J., Kent-Walsh, J., & Hickman, S. (2008). The impacts of aided AAC interventions on AAC use, speech, and symbolic gestures. *Seminars in Speech and Language, 29*, 101-111.

Binger, C., & Kent-Walsh, J. (2008). *Supporting turn-taking in AAC: Instruction for SLPs, parents, and peers.* Paper presented at the annual conference of the American Speech-Language-Hearing Association, Chicago, IL.

Binger, C., Kent-Walsh, J., Berens, J., Del Campo, S., & Rivera, D. (2008). Teaching Latino parents to support the multi-symbol message productions of their children who require AAC. *Augmentative and Alternative Communication, 24*(323-338).

Binger, C., Kent-Walsh, J., Ewing, C., & Taylor, S. (in press). Teaching educational assistants to facilitate multi-symbol message productions of young students who require AAC. *American Journal of Speech-Language Pathology.*

Binger, C., & Light, J. (2006). Demographics of preschoolers who require AAC. *Speech, Language, and Hearing Services in Schools, 37*, 200-208.

Blackstone, S. (1994). The purpose of AAC assessment. *Augmentative Communication News, 7*, 2-3.

Blockberger, S., & Sutton, A. (2003). Toward linguistic competence: The language experiences and knowledge of children with extremely limited speech. In J. Light & D. Beukelman & J. Reichle (Eds.), *Communicative competence for individuals who use augmentative and alternative communication.* Baltimore: Paul H. Brookes Publishing Co.

Downing, J., & Falvey, M. (2005). *Teaching communication skills to students with severe disabilities* (2 ed.). Baltimore, MD: Paul H. Brookes Publishing Co.

Giangreco, M. F. (1990). Making related service decisions for students with severe disabilities: Roles, criteria, and authority. *Journal of the Association for Persons with Severe Handicaps, 13*, 22-31.

Glennen, S. L., & DeCoste, D. C. (1997). *Handbook of augmentative and alternative communication*. San Diego, CA: Singular Publishing Group, Inc.

Kent-Walsh, J., & McNaughton, D. (2005). Communication partner instruction in AAC: Present practices and future directions. Augmentative and Alternative Communication, 21, 195-204.

Kent-Walsh, J., Stark, C., & Binger, C. (2008). Tales from school trenches: AAC service-delivery and professional expertise. *Seminars in Speech and Langauge, 29*, 146-154.

Light, J. (1989). Toward a definition of communicative competence for individuals using augmentative and alternative communication. *Augmentative and Alternative Communication, 5*, 137-144.

Light, J., & Binger, C. (1998). *Building communicative competence with individuals who use augmentative and alternative communication*. Baltimore: Paul H. Brookes Publishing Co.

Lloyd, L., Fuller, D., & Arvidson, H. (1997). *Augmentative and alternative communication: A handbook of principles and practices*. Boston: Allyn & Bacon.

Millar, D., Light, J. C., & Schlosser, R. W. (2006). The impact of augmentative and alternative communication on the speech production of individuals with developmental disabilities: A research review. *Journal of Speech, Language, and Hearing Research, 49*, 248-264.

National Joint Committee for the Communication Needs of Persons with Severe Disabilities. (1992). Guidelines for meeting the communication needs of persons with severe disabilities. *Asha, 34*(Suppl. 7), 2-3.

Owens, R. E. J. (2008). *Language development: An introduction* (7 ed.). Needham Heights, MA: Allyn & Bacon.

Rosa-Lugo, L. I., & Kent-Walsh, J. (2008). Effects of parent instruction on communicative turns of Latino children using AAC during storybook reading. Communication Disorders Quarterly, 30, 49-61.

Sansosti, F., Powell-Smith, K., & Kincaid, D. (2004). A research synthesis of social story interventions for children with autism spectrum disorders. *Focus on Autism and Other Developmental Disabilities, 19*, 194-204.

Soto, G., Müller, E., Hunt, P., & Goetz, L. (2001). Critical issues in the inclusion of students who use augmentative and alternative communication: An educational team perspective. *Augmentative and Alternative Communication, 17*, 62-72.

Tech Act. (1988). Assistive Technology. Retrieved from http://standards.gov/standards_gov/assistiveTechnology.cfm.

Yoder, P., & Stone, W. L. (2006). A randomized comparison of the effect of two prelinguistic communication interventions on the acquisition of spoken communication in preschoolers with ASD. *Journal of Speech, Language, and Hearing Research, 49*, 698-711.

Zangari, C., & Soto, G. (2009). *Practically speaking: Language, literacy, and academic development for students with AAC needs*. Baltimore: Paul H. Brookes Publishing Co.